DR. SEBI ULTIMATE JUICING RECIPES FOR CANCER

Harness Nature's Power with Potent Elixirs. Unleash the Healing Potential, Supercharge Your Body, and Triumph Over Cancer

CW01497753

MIGUEL T. BEATON

COPYRIGHT © 2023 BY MIGUEL T. BEATON

UNDERSTANDING DR. SEBI'S APPROACH

Alfredo Darrington Bowman, better known as Dr. Sebi, was a self-taught herbalist and healer from Honduras. His concentration on natural, plant-based medicines and his holistic approach to health helped him become well-known. The foundation of Dr. Sebi's theory is the idea that keeping the body's environment alkaline is essential for both treating and preventing a wide range of illnesses. In addition to nutritional advice, his teachings cover the use of herbs and lifestyle modifications that promote general wellbeing.

Alkaline Diet Fundamentals

Dr. Sebi's philosophy revolves around the idea of an alkaline diet. The foundation of the alkaline diet is the hypothesis that some meals leave an alkaline residue in the body after they are digested. Dr. Sebi asserts that maintaining an alkaline environment is critical to the body's healthy operation and the avoidance of illness. The diet is mostly plant-based, with a focus on raw fruits and vegetables, along with grains, nuts, and seeds.

Foods were divided into three primary categories by Dr. Sebi: hybrid, acidic, and alkaline. Because they are said to be able to increase the body's pH levels and foster an environment that inhibits the growth of diseases, alkaline meals are advised. Leafy greens, fruits, nuts, and grains are a few of these. Conversely, foods high in acidity, such meat, dairy, and processed foods, should be avoided because they may have a role in the onset of some illnesses. Dr. Sebi claims that hybrid foods are unnatural mixes that ought to be avoided.

The Function of Herbs in Dr. Sebi's Suggestions

A key component of Dr. Sebi's approach to wellness is herbal therapy. He promoted the use of particular plants to nourish and cleanse the body. According to Dr. Sebi, herbs possess inherent therapeutic qualities that can help the body's natural healing processes and address a range of health problems.

Dr. Sebi frequently suggests burdock root, sarsaparilla, dandelion, and chaparral as plants. These plants are said to help with blood purification, body detoxification, and general wellbeing. It's crucial to remember that although herbal medicines have been used for centuries in traditional medicine, there may not be enough scientific proof to support their effectiveness when used in conjunction with Dr. Sebi's particular prescriptions.

Juicing's Significance in Cancer Prevention

The advantages of juicing for establishing and preserving an alkaline condition in the body were emphasized by Dr. Sebi.

Juicing is the process of removing the fibrous pulp from fruits and vegetables and extracting their liquid content. Dr. Sebi claims that drinking fresh juices can supply the body with concentrated forms of vital nutrients, facilitating improved absorption and use.

Juicing, according to Dr. Sebi, is an effective way to alkalize the body and make it less conducive to the growth of cancer cells. Alkaline fruits like berries and melons, as well as green leafy vegetables like spinach and kale, are frequently suggested for juicing in Dr. Sebi's method.

The specific assertion that juicing can prevent cancer or produce an environment hostile to cancer cells may not have strong scientific support, despite the fact that there is research supporting the health advantages of eating fruits and vegetables. People should approach these kinds of statements with a skeptical perspective and seek the opinion of medical specialists for specific guidance.

Smoothies' Health Benefits for Your Diet

Dr. Sebi also recommended smoothies as a way to include more fruits and vegetables in one's diet. Generally, whole fruits and vegetables—including their fiber content—are blended to create smoothies. Compared to juicing, this approach preserves the healthy fiber and offers a distinct nutritional profile.

Smoothies provide an easy method to get multiple nutrient-dense foods in one serving. For general health and well-being, Dr. Sebi suggested adding alkaline fruits and vegetables to smoothies. People can alter the components in their smoothies to suit their dietary requirements and taste preferences.

Smoothie fiber helps support healthy digestion and may help control blood sugar levels. Furthermore, adding nuts and seeds to smoothies might supply necessary proteins and lipids. It is important to remember, nevertheless, that the overall health effects of smoothies depend on the particular ingredients that are used as well as the overall composition of the diet.

Dr. Sebi bases his approach to health on the ideas that an alkaline environment may be maintained in the body by following a plant-based diet, using herbal medicines, and changing one's lifestyle. Even if his teachings have become more well-known, it's important to examine them critically and recognize that there isn't enough scientific data to back some of the more specific claims.

The alkaline diet fits with general guidelines for a healthy diet because it emphasizes plant-based foods and discourages the consumption of some acidic and hybrid foods. The rigorous division of foods into groups based on their acidity, alkalinity, and hybridity, however, might oversimplify the complexities of nutritional research.

Although traditional medicine has a long history of using herbs to promote health, Dr. Sebi's exact recommendations may not have received thorough scientific validation for their effectiveness in his particular method.

Smoothies and juices are easy ways to up your intake of fruits and vegetables, but they shouldn't be seen as stand-alone treatments for particular ailments; rather, they should be seen as supplements to a balanced diet.

In conclusion, people who are interested in implementing Dr. Sebi's strategy ought to do it mindfully, taking into account their particular health requirements and seeking the advice of medical specialists for tailored advice. Furthermore, it's critical to understand that while some aspects of Dr. Sebi's philosophy can be consistent with broad guidelines for healthy living, some of his specific assertions do not have strong scientific backing.

CHAPTER ONE

ALKALINE FRUITS TO PREVENT CANCER

There has been a lot of study and debate on the connection between nutrition and cancer prevention. A diet high in specific nutrients and antioxidants may help reduce the risk of cancer, even if no one meal or combination of foods may ensure the disease's prevention. The alkaline diet, which stresses the consumption of foods that generate an alkaline environment, such as fruits, is one dietary strategy that has gained popularity in this context. We explore the world of alkaline fruits and their possible significance in preventing cancer in this investigation.

Examining Fruits High in Alkali:

Fruits that leave an alkaline residue in the body after metabolism are known as alkaline fruits. Proponents of the alkaline diet, such as Dr. Sebi, contend that keeping the body's environment alkaline can help fend against illnesses like cancer. There is general agreement regarding the health advantages of eating fruits as part of a balanced diet, even though there may not be enough scientific data to support this particular claim.

Typical alkaline fruit varieties are:

1.Berries: Packed with fiber, vitamins, and antioxidants, berries are a great option for general health. Because they neutralize free radicals, which can harm cells and contribute to the development of cancer, antioxidants like the anthocyanins present in blueberries and raspberries have been linked to the prevention of cancer. By including a range of berries in your diet, you may support your body's natural defense mechanisms with a spectrum of nutrients.

How to Include Berries in Your Diet:

Berries are a tasty and wholesome option to improve your consumption of alkaline foods in your diet. Think about the following concepts:

• Smoothies: For a hydrating and nutrient-dense smoothie, blend a variety of berries with an alkaline vegetable basis, such as spinach or kale.

• Snacking: Berries provide a filling and wholesome snack either eaten on their own or combined with nuts.

• Salads: for berries to salads to for extra antioxidants and a taste boost.

2.The Anti-Cancer Properties of Citrus Fruits: Citrus fruits, such as grapefruits, oranges, lemons, and limes, are renowned for having a high vitamin C concentration. Antioxidant vitamin C is essential for bolstering the immune system and shielding cells from harm. Citrus fruits' acidity may seem to go against the alkaline diet, yet after they are metabolized, they have an alkalizing impact on the body.

Studies indicate that vitamin C may offer protection against specific cancer forms. Research has examined its possible function in lowering the risk of breast and colorectal cancers, for instance. Citrus fruits also have other bioactive substances, like flavonoids, which enhance their anti-cancer capabilities.

Including Fruits with Citrus in Your Diet:

• Fresh Juices: To produce your own juices, squeeze fresh citrus fruits. If desired, dilute with water to lessen acidity.

• Salad Dressings: To make tasty, alkaline salad dressings, use citrus fruits.

• Snacking: As a cool and hydrated snack, eat citrus fruits.

3.Melons for Hydration and Nutrients: Melons, such as honeydew, cantaloupe, and watermelon, are not only nutrient- and hydration-dense but also delicious. These fruits include vital vitamins, minerals, and antioxidants and are alkaline-forming. Particularly watermelon is renowned for having a high water content, which helps with hydration—a vital component of good health.

Studies have looked into the possibility that lycopene, which is found in watermelon, can lower the chance of developing some cancers, such as prostate cancer. Lycopene, a potent antioxidant, is responsible for the vivid red color of watermelon.

How to Include Melons in Your Diet:

• Fruit Salads: To make a cool and hydrating fruit salad, mix melons with other alkaline fruits.

• Smoothies: For a nutrient-rich smoothie, blend melon pieces with berries and leafy greens.

• Hydration: Watermelon slices are a refreshing snack, particularly in hot weather.

4.Tropical Fruits with Healing Properties: In addition to offering a variety of health advantages, tropical fruits like papaya, mango, and pineapple also add deliciousness. In addition to being alkaline-forming, these fruits are a great source of vitamins, antioxidants, and enzymes that support general health.

Papain, an enzyme recognized for its digestive qualities, is found in papayas. Health in general and the absorption of nutrients depend on proper digestion. Papaya is also a great source of antioxidants, folate, and vitamin C, all of which help the body's defense processes.

How to Include Tropical Fruits in Your Diet:

• Fruit Salsas: To go with grilled food or as a stand-alone snack, make salsas using a variety of tropical fruits.

• Desserts: Tropical fruits make a tasty and wholesome dessert when consumed in moderation.

• Smoothie Bowls: For a filling and alkaline-rich breakfast, blend tropical fruits and sprinkle nuts and seeds on top.

In summary:

Despite the fact that the alkaline diet—which places a strong emphasis on alkaline fruits—has grown in popularity due to its possible health advantages, it's crucial to have a balanced viewpoint. All things considered, fruits provide a wealth of nutrients, antioxidants, and fiber that support general health and may even help prevent cancer.

A holistic approach to health can benefit from including a range of alkaline fruits in your diet as well as from keeping an eating pattern that is varied and well-balanced. For individualized nutritional advice, it's best to speak with medical professionals, particularly for those who already have health issues.

To sum up, adding alkaline fruits to a well-rounded diet can enhance its flavor and healthfulness and strengthen the body's natural defenses against illnesses like cancer. Examples of these fruits are berries, citrus fruits, melons, and tropical fruits.

CHAPTER TWO

HERBAL MEDICINES AND THEIR IMPORTANCE

Herbal medicine has long been used to treat illnesses and enhance wellbeing in human history. Many traditional medical systems have acknowledged the therapeutic benefits of many plants, including Ayurveda, Traditional Chinese Medicine, and Native American herbalism. A rising corpus of research examining the possible health advantages of various plants has led to a renaissance of interest in herbal medicine in the modern day. This investigation explores the importance of medicinal herbs, classifying them according to their functions in enhancing immunity, supporting cellular health, reducing inflammation, and enhancing general health.

Herbs to Strengthen Your Immune System:

The immune system is essential for protecting the body from illnesses and infections. Herbal remedies have long been utilized to strengthen the body's defenses against disease and improve immunological function.

1.Native to North America, echinacea is a flowering plant. Native American cultures have long utilized it for its immune-boosting qualities. It is thought that echinacea increases the formation of white blood cells, which are vital for warding against illnesses. Additionally, it contains substances that have antioxidant and anti-inflammatory properties.

2.Astragalus: Known for bolstering the immune system, astragalus is prized in traditional Chinese medicine. It is thought to improve general vigor and strengthen the body's defenses against illnesses. Polysaccharides and flavonoids included in astragalus aid in enhancing the immune system.

3.Garlic: Throughout history, people have utilized garlic's therapeutic qualities. Allicin, a substance with antibacterial and immune-boosting qualities, is present in it. It is thought that garlic increases immune cell activity, which may aid in both infection prevention and treatment.

Including Herbs That Boost the Immune System in Your Daily Routine:

• Herbal Teas: Use astragalus and echinacea, two herbs that strengthen the immune system, to make teas. Regularly consume these teas to boost your immune system.

• Supplements: Take into account taking herbal supplements that contain immune-boosting herbs, but check the amounts with a medical practitioner.

• Culinary Use: Use garlic in your food preparation to reap the flavor and immunological-boosting benefits.

Herbs that Detoxify for Cellular Health:

People who lead modern lifestyles are exposed to a variety of environmental contaminants, pollutants, and processed foods, all of which can build up in the body. It is thought that detoxifying herbs aid in the body's natural detoxification processes, enhancing general wellbeing and cellular health.

1.Dandelion Root: For centuries, people have utilized dandelion root as a liver tonic. The liver is a vital organ in the detoxification process, and dandelion root is thought to promote liver health. It might facilitate the body's removal of toxins.

2.Another herb with a reputation for shielding the liver is milk thistle. It contains a substance known as silymarin, which has anti-inflammatory and antioxidant properties. It is thought that silymarin aids in liver cell regeneration and facilitates detoxification.

3.Burdock Root: Because of its blood-cleansing qualities, burdock root is frequently employed in traditional medicine. It is thought to support clear skin and aid in the lymphatic system's removal of pollutants. Additionally, burdock root possesses anti-inflammatory and antioxidant properties.

Including Herbs for Detoxification in Your Daily Routine:

• Herbal Infusions: Use burdock, milk thistle, and dandelion root to make herbal infusions. Regularly consume these infusions as part of a detoxification regimen.

• Herbal Supplements: Take into account taking herbal supplements that contain cleansing herbs, but make sure you speak with a doctor about how to use them properly.

• Use in Cooking: Include purifying herbs in your dishes. For instance, include burdock root into stir-fries or add dandelion leaves to salads.

Herbs Anti-Inflammatory in the Prevention of Cancer:

Cancer is among the many disorders that have been connected to chronic inflammation. Herbs that inhibit inflammation are thought to help control the body's inflammatory response and lower the chance of developing chronic illnesses.

1.Turmeric: Curcumin, the key ingredient in turmeric, is a well-known herb having anti-inflammatory properties. Curcumin's ability to prevent and treat a variety of malignancies has been thoroughly investigated. It functions by displaying antioxidant qualities and blocking inflammatory pathways.

2.Ginger: Another herb that has antioxidant and anti-inflammatory properties is ginger. It possesses gingerol, a bioactive substance that has been researched for possible cancer prevention. Inflammation and oxidative stress in the body may be lessened by ginger.

3.Green Tea: Green tea contains a lot of polyphenols, especially catechins, which have antioxidant and anti-inflammatory qualities. Green tea's epigallocatechin gallate (EGCG), a catechin, has been researched for its ability to stop cancer cells from growing.

Including Herbs That Reduce Inflammation in Your Daily Routine:

• Golden Milk: Make golden milk with other warming spices and turmeric. This classic Ayurvedic drink can be a calming and anti-inflammatory supplement to your daily regimen.

• Herbal Teas: Savor teas prepared with anti-inflammatory herbs, such as green tea and ginger. You can eat these every day to help maintain general health.

• Spice Blends: When making spice blends for cooking, include ginger and turmeric. Try adding these herbs to a range of different recipes.

Adaptogenic Plants for General Health:

Herbs classified as adaptogens are thought to support the body's ability to adjust to stress and preserve equilibrium. These plants have long been used to promote general mental and physical health.

1.Ashwagandha: Traditionally used in Ayurvedic medicine, ashwagandha is an adaptogenic plant. By regulating the stress response and bolstering the adrenal glands, it's thought to assist the body in handling stress. Additionally, ashwagandha may have anti-inflammatory and immune-modulating properties.

2.Rhodiola Rosea: Traditionally, Scandinavian and Russian medicine has utilized rhodiola, an adaptogen. It is thought to lessen fatigue, increase mental performance, and strengthen resilience to stress. Antioxidant qualities may also be present in rhodiola.

3.Holy Basil (Tulsi): In Ayurveda, holy basil, also known as tulsi, is revered as a sacred herb. It is said to contain adaptogenic qualities that make the body more capable of handling stress. Additionally, holy basil may have immune-modulating and anti-inflammatory properties.

Adding Adaptogenic Herbs to Your Daily Routine:

• Herbal Infusions: Use adaptogenic herbs such as holy basil, rhodiola, and ashwagandha to make infusions. You can drink these as soothing teas.

• Supplements: Take into account adaptogenic herbal supplements; however, for proper usage, seek medical advice.

• Culinary Use: Add adaptogenic herbs as garnishes or in cooking. For instance, infuse warm beverages with ashwagandha or garnish dishes with fresh leaves of holy basil.

In both traditional and modern approaches to health and well-being, healing herbs are important. Although the precise workings and effectiveness of these herbs may differ, their traditional application and growing scientific attention underscore their potential benefits for a range of health issues.

Including medicinal herbs in your regimen can be a comprehensive approach to bolster immune system performance, encourage cellular health, avert inflammation, and improve general wellbeing. But it's important to use caution while using herbal medicines and to seek medical advice as needed, particularly if you have a history of health issues or are taking medication.

In conclusion, the various therapeutic qualities of healing herbs are what make them significant, and incorporating them into a diversified and balanced lifestyle can be an important part of an all-encompassing strategy for health and wellbeing.

CHAPTER THREE

STRONG JUICES TO COMBAT CANCER

Research and interest in the role of nutrition in managing and preventing cancer are on the rise. Although there isn't a single food or drink that might prevent or cure cancer, some nutrient-rich juices—especially those prepared from vegetables—are being researched for their possible advantages. We'll talk about how to make nutrient-rich vegetable juices and how they affect cancer cells in this discussion. We'll also talk about how root veggies help prevent cancer, the advantages of making juices with herbs included, and how important it is to balance savory and sweet liquids for both flavor and health.

Making Vegetable Juices High in Nutrients:

Vegetable juices, which are a powerful source of vitamins, minerals, antioxidants, and phytochemicals, are a great method to concentrate the nutritional value of a range of vegetables. Vegetables with proven anti-cancer qualities are generally the focus when it comes to cancer prevention.

1.Cruciferous Vegetables: Cruciferous vegetables, which include Brussels sprouts, broccoli, kale, and cabbage, are well-known for their ability to prevent cancer. They contain substances that have been researched for their capacity to prevent the formation of cancer cells and support the body's detoxification process, such as sulforaphane and indole-3-carbinol.

Juice Tip: Blend kale, broccoli, celery, and cucumber to make a nutrient-rich juice. For flavor and to boost your vitamin C intake, squeeze in some lemon juice.

2.Leafy Greens: High in vitamins, minerals, and antioxidants, leafy greens include collard greens, spinach, and Swiss chard. These greens' high chlorophyll content could be a factor in their possible anti-cancer qualities.

Juice Tip: Combine spinach, cucumber, green apple, and a dash of mint for freshness to create a brilliant green juice.

3.Carotenoids-Rich Vegetables: Carotenoids-rich vegetables, such bell peppers, sweet potatoes, and carrots, offer a vibrant range of nutrients. Beta-carotene is one of the carotenoids that have antioxidant qualities that may help shield cells from harm.

Juice Tip: Blend carrots, sweet potatoes, and bell peppers to make a visually beautiful and nutrient-rich juice. A little of ginger can be added for even more flavor.

Green Juices' Effect on Cancer Cells:

Green juices, which frequently include a range of leafy greens and other green vegetables, have become more and more well-liked due to their possible health advantages, which include preventing cancer. The anti-cancer benefits of green vegetables are attributed to their chlorophyll, vitamins, and minerals content.

1.Chlorophyll and Detoxification: Research has been done on the possibility that chlorophyll, the green pigment found in plants, can help with detoxification. It might assist the liver, an essential organ for detoxification, and aid the body in getting rid of pollutants. A less contaminated, more hygienic environment within the body could lower the risk of cancer.

Juice Tip: Add greens high in chlorophyll, such as spinach, kale, and wheatgrass, to your green juices. Squeeze in some lemon to help with cleansing.

2.Antioxidants and Cell Protection: The body uses antioxidants found in green vegetables to counteract free radicals. Unstable chemicals called free radicals have the potential to harm cells and advance the onset of cancer. Antioxidants aid in defending cells against such harm.

Juice Tip: To increase antioxidant content, blend several green veggies together, such cucumber, celery, and green apples. Add some herbs, such as parsley, to enhance the antioxidant content even further.

Root Vegetables and Their Potential to Fight Cancer:

In addition to having rich nutrient profiles and earthy flavors, root vegetables can help prevent cancer. They have a variety of antioxidants and phytochemicals that support general health and may help prevent cancer.

1.Beets: Studies have examined the possible anti-inflammatory and antioxidant properties of betalains, which are abundant in beets. Additionally, beets' pigment betanin may have anti-cancer qualities.

Juice Tip: For a refreshing twist, blend beets with carrots, apples, and a dash of lemon to create a colorful beet juice.

2.Ginger: A rhizome with strong anti-inflammatory and antioxidant qualities, ginger is not a root vegetable. It possesses gingerol, which has been researched for possible use in treating and preventing cancer of different kinds.

Juice Tip: For flavor and possible health advantages, use a small piece of fresh ginger in your vegetable juices.

3.Turmeric: Turmeric's anti-inflammatory and antioxidant qualities are attributed to its active ingredient, curcumin. Research indicates that curcumin may possess anti-cancer properties by impeding the proliferation of cancerous cells.

Juice Tip: To improve the absorption of curcumin, blend turmeric, carrots, oranges, and a small amount of black pepper into a golden-hued juice.

Juices with Herb Infusions for Maximum Benefits:

In addition to adding flavor to juices, herbs offer special compounds that may have health advantages. You can improve the nutritional profile of your juices and give yourself extra support for general wellbeing by adding herbs to them.

1.Parsley: Packed with vitamins, minerals, and chlorophyll. Flavonoids, which have antioxidant qualities, are also present in it. Juices with parsley in them have the potential to be more detoxifying and cell-protective.

Juice Tip: To enhance the nutritional value and freshness of green juices, add a handful of fresh parsley.

2.Basil: Flavonoids and essential oils are among the substances in basil that may have anti-cancer effects. It also gives juices a delicious flavor boost.

Juice Tip: Add some basil to your juices to give them a flavor boost. For a pleasant cocktail, try mixing it with bell peppers, tomatoes, and cucumbers.

3.Coriander, or cilantro, is a leafy green that has been examined for its ability to aid in detoxifying. It is high in antioxidants. Adding cilantro to your juices could improve the health of your cells in general.

Juice Tip: For a nutrient-rich and purifying juice, blend cilantro with cucumber and celery or other green vegetables.

Juicing to Balance Sweet and Savory Flavors for Health and Taste:

While adding veggies to juices is often the focus due to their health advantages, it's crucial to balance the flavors of salty and sweet ingredients to create long-lasting, pleasurable juices.

1.Sweet Juices: Fruits that naturally contribute sweetness to juices, such as apples, berries, and citrus fruits, also include vital vitamins and antioxidants. Though it's important to watch how much sugar you eat, fruit sweetness can help make veggie juices taste better.

Juice Tip: Use leafy greens, cucumber, and celery to counterbalance sweetness in your juice. Instead of depending too much on fruit sugars, try enhancing the flavor with a squeeze of lemon.

2.Savory Juices: Dark leafy greens, tomatoes, and bell peppers are among the vegetables that give juices a powerful and savory flavor. These veggies provide a variety of nutrients, such as antioxidants, minerals, and vitamins.

Juice Tip: Try blending tomatoes, bell peppers, celery, and a small amount of garlic for a savory twist when experimenting with savory juices.

3.Hydration and Flavor: Adding hydrating components to the juice, such as cucumber and celery, not only makes it more hydrated but also enhances its flavor. Staying hydrated is crucial for maintaining the health of cells and can enhance the nutrients included in the juice.

Juice Tip: Start your juices with cucumber and add different vegetables and herbs to build tastes.

Juices with potent anti-cancer properties can be a great complement to any health-conscious diet. Juices that are both beneficial and delightful are made from a blend of nutrient-rich vegetables, greens, root vegetables, herbs, and a well-balanced combination of sweet and savory flavors.

It's crucial to remember that while there is proof that some meals may help prevent cancer, each person's reaction may be different. Juices should also be seen as an integral component of a holistic approach to health, supporting other healthy lifestyle behaviors such as a balanced diet and frequent exercise.

Trying out various concoctions, tastes, and components enables personalization according to dietary requirements and tastes. It's wise to speak with medical professionals before making any dietary changes, as this is especially important for people with pre-existing medical disorders or those receiving cancer treatment.

In summary, carefully choosing elements with proven or possible cancer-fighting qualities is necessary to create nutrient-rich vegetable juices. These juices, which include cruciferous and root vegetables, herbs, and a harmony of sweet and savory flavors, can add taste and health to a wellness-oriented way of living.

CHAPTER FOUR

SMOOTHIES FOR CELLULAR NOURISHMENT

Smoothies are now a common and practical way to add a range of nutrients to our meals, giving our cells a tasty and effective approach to be nourished. We will examine the process of creating nutrient-dense smoothies that support cellular sustenance in this investigation. We'll look at many smoothie types, such as Green Elixir Smoothies for cleansing, Berry Blast Smoothies for a tasty twist, Tropical Paradise Smoothies for a unique taste, and the use of herbal infusions for medicinal purposes.

Making Smoothies Packed with Nutrients:

Smoothies packed with nutrients are made possible by carefully choosing ingredients that provide an array of vitamins, minerals, antioxidants, and other health-promoting substances. The following are crucial elements to take into account when creating nutrient-dense smoothies for cellular hydration:

1. Leafy Greens: High in antioxidants, minerals (including iron and calcium), and vitamins (like A, C, and K), leafy greens include spinach, kale, and Swiss chard. These greens provide your smoothies a strong nutritional base while also supporting general cellular health.

2. Berries: Rich in anthocyanins, which are powerful antioxidants, berries including raspberries, strawberries, and blueberries are also delightful. Numerous health advantages, such as promoting cellular health and preventing oxidative stress, have been linked to these substances.

3. Healthy Fats: You may improve the nutritional profile of your smoothies by include sources of healthy fats like avocados, chia seeds, and flaxseeds. Both cellular function and the absorption of fat-soluble vitamins depend heavily on healthy lipids.

4. Protein Sources: Consuming foods high in protein, such as protein powder, Greek yogurt, or almond butter, can aid in the regeneration and repair of cells.

Protein can help with general cellular nourishment and is necessary for the construction and repair of tissues. You can include protein in your smoothies.

5. Liquid basis: For your smoothies, pick a nutrient-dense liquid basis like green tea, coconut water, or almond milk. These choices offer extra vitamins, minerals, and water in addition to taste.

6. Superfoods: For an additional nutritional boost, think about including superfoods like acai berries, chlorella, or spirulina. Superfoods are frequently abundant in vitamins, minerals, and antioxidants that support cellular health.

Recipes for Berry Blast Smoothies:

Berries are a great option for improving cellular health because they are not only delicious but also a great source of vitamins and antioxidants. Try these two recipes for Berry Blast Smoothies:

1. Berry Citrus Burst: 1/2 cup Greek yogurt; 1 cup mixed berries (strawberries, raspberries, and blueberries).

• One-half orange, peeled; • One-cup coconut water; • One tablespoon chia seeds; • Optional ice cubes

Directions: Process until smooth, blending all ingredients. If necessary, add extra coconut water to adjust consistency.

2. Antioxidant Powerhouse Smoothie: 1 cup blackberries, 1/2 cup pomegranate

seeds, 1/2 cup frozen or pureed acai berries, 1 tablespoon almond butter, 1 cup almond milk, and 1 teaspoon honey (optional)

Directions: Process all ingredients in a blender until fully blended. If desired, add honey to sweeten.

Smoothies with Green Elixir for Detoxification:

Smoothies with green elixir are made to aid the body's detoxification processes, encouraging cellular purification and general health. You may make your own Green Elixir Smoothies using these two recipes:

1. Detox Green Goddess: 1 teaspoon spirulina powder; 2 cups spinach; 1/2

peeled cucumber; 1/2 avocado; 1/2 juiced lemon;

• One cup of coconut water • Optional ice cubes

Directions: Process until smooth, blending all ingredients. If necessary, add extra coconut water to adjust consistency.

2. Cucumber Mint Elixir for Cleaning: 1 cup kale; 1/2 peeled cucumber; 1/4 cup fresh mint leaves; 1/2 cored green apple; 1 tablespoon chia seeds; 1 cup cooled green tea; optional ice cubes

Directions: Process all ingredients in a blender until fully blended. If you like a thinner consistency, add extra green tea.

Tropical Paradise Drinks with a Tasty Hint:

Tropical Paradise Smoothies offer a multitude of nutrients and a taste explosion of unique flavors. To take your taste senses to a tropical oasis, try these two recipes:

1. Mango Pineapple Bliss: 1/2 cup pineapple chunks, 1/2 cup fresh or frozen mango pieces, 1/2 banana, and 1/2 cup Greek yogurt

• One-ton flaxseeds; one-cup coconut water; optional ice cubes

Directions: Process until smooth, blending all ingredients. If necessary, add extra coconut water to adjust consistency.

2. Coconut Kiwi Delight consists of the following ingredients: 1 cup peeled and sliced kiwi; 1/2 cup coconut milk; 1/2

avocado; 1 tablespoon hemp seeds; 1 teaspoon lime juice; 1 cup water or coconut water; and optional ice cubes.

Directions: Process all ingredients in a blender until fully blended. If desired, adjust sweetness with agave or honey.

Smoothie Infusions with Herbal Infusions for Healing Properties:

Herbal infusions can give your smoothies a therapeutic touch by adding taste and possibly even health benefits. Here are two smoothie recipes with herbal infusions to try:

1. Minty Green Revitalizer: 2 cups spinach; 1/2 peeled cucumber; 1/4 cup fresh mint leaves; 1/2 cored green apple; ½ tablespoon chia seeds; 1 cup chilled mint tea

• Ice cubes, if desired

Directions: Process until smooth, blending all ingredients. If necessary, add extra mint tea to adjust consistency.

2. Serenity Lavender Berry:

• 1/2 cup Greek yogurt; 1 cup mixed berries (strawberries, raspberries, and blueberries)

• 1/2 teaspoon of culinary-grade dried lavender buds; 1 tablespoon of flaxseeds; and 1 cup of chilled chamomile tea

• Ice cubes, if desired

Directions: Process all ingredients in a blender until fully blended. If desired, adjust sweetness with honey.

In summary, smoothies provide an adaptable platform for blending nutrient-rich mixtures that facilitate cellular hydration. Choosing components that support general wellbeing is crucial, whether you go for Berry Blast Smoothies, Green Elixir Smoothies, Tropical Paradise Smoothies, or try out herbal infusions.

Smoothies that are full of flavor and provide a range of vitamins, minerals, antioxidants, and other bioactive compounds that are critical for cellular health can be made by mixing in a variety of fruits, vegetables, greens, and other superfoods.

Smoothies are a fun and easy method to add extra nutrients to your diet for the best possible cellular nourishment. Consult a healthcare provider before making any dietary adjustments, as is the case with those who have pre-existing medical conditions or special dietary needs.

To sum up, learn how to make nutrient-dense smoothies and use them to enhance your general health and cellular health. Try a variety of foods, flavors, and textures to find combinations that will delight your taste buds and nourish your cells.

CHAPTER FIVE

PRACTICAL ADVICE FOR INCLUDING DR. SEBI'S RECIPES

The dietary philosophy of Dr. Sebi places a strong emphasis on an alkaline diet that is composed primarily of whole, plant-based foods that promote overall health and wellbeing. Adopting this lifestyle can result in positive results, but it needs thoughtful planning, preparation, and selection of foods. We'll talk about doable strategies for implementing Dr. Sebi's recipes into your daily routine in this session. We'll cover topics like making the switch to an alkaline lifestyle, grocery shopping, meal planning, maintaining a consistent juice and smoothie routine, and mindful eating for overall health.

Changing Your Lifestyle to an Alkaline One:

1. Become knowledgeable: Spend some time learning the foundational ideas of Dr. Sebi's method before committing to an alkaline lifestyle. Discover the differences between foods that are alkaline and acidic, the value of plant-based nutrition, and the possible advantages of adhering to this dietary philosophy.

2. Gradual Change: Consider making modest modifications so your body can adjust rather than making big changes all at once. Increase the amount of alkaline

foods in your meals at first, and then progressively cut back on acidic ones. This strategy might lessen the likelihood of detoxification symptoms.

3. Water Is Important: Stress how crucial staying hydrated is to preserving an alkaline balance. For a cool, alkalizing beverage, choose alkaline water or water with lemon added. Maintaining adequate hydration promotes general health and helps the body flush out impurities.

Purchasing Food to Support Dr. Sebi's Diet:

1. Emphasis on entire, Plant-centered Foods: Eating a diet centered on entire, plant-based foods is encouraged by Dr. Sebi. Give organic produce, grains, beans, and fruits first priority. To

optimize nutritional value and reduce exposure to chemicals and pesticides, use fresh produce.

2. Alkaline Staples: Assemble an assortment of nuts and seeds, quinoa, wild rice, spelt, and chickpeas in your cupboard. Several recipes that have been approved by Dr. Sebi start with these ingredients.

3. Herbs and spices: Investigate a range of spices and herbs that complement Dr. Sebi's suggestions. Use herbs and spices such as sage, thyme, oregano, and cayenne pepper to add flavor to your food without making it lose its alkalinity.

4. Make a Variety Plan: To guarantee a wide range of nutrients, Dr. Sebi's diet recommends a varied assortment of

meals. If you want to maintain an intriguing and nutritionally balanced diet, make sure your meals feature a range of colors, textures, and flavors.

Organizing Meals and Getting Ready for Success:

1. Batch Cooking: To make meal preparation easier, cook essentials like grains, beans, and vegetables in large quantities. It is simpler to put up well-balanced meals throughout the week when these ingredients are on hand, which saves time and guarantees that the alkaline diet is followed.

2. Prepare and Clean Produce: Set aside time to prepare, wash, and chop fruits and vegetables. When wholesome selections are easily accessible, this

preparation not only saves time during the week but also enhances the likelihood of selecting healthy snacks.

3. Prepare Balanced Meals: Arrange your meals such that they contain an equal amount of alkaline foods, a source of protein (such as lentils or chickpeas), and healthy fats (such as avocado, almonds, or seeds). This harmony makes it possible for you to adhere to Dr. Sebi's recommendations while still getting the nourishment you need.

4. Look Into New Recipes: Try out some new dishes that follow Dr. Sebi's guidelines to make your meals interesting. Alkaline meals can be made in a variety of tasty and inventive ways, from salads and soups to plant-based protein dishes.

Maintaining Your Smoothie and Juicing Habits:

Invest in a Good Juicer and Blender: Purchasing a good juicer and blender is essential if you want to follow Dr. Sebi's advice to the letter. These kitchen tools are necessary to make nutrient-rich smoothies and juices, which will make it easier for you to include alkaline foods in your regular diet.

2. Plan Your Juicing Schedule: To help juicing become a habit that lasts, set up a regular timetable. Setting aside time to juice will help you stick to the habit, whether it's as a morning ritual or an afternoon energy boost.

3. Vary Up Your Ingredients: Try making juices and smoothies with different

fruits, veggies, and herbs. The components that Dr. Sebi has approved have a wide range of tastes and nutritional advantages. Including a variety of ingredients guarantees a wide range of nutrients and helps avoid taste fatigue.

4. Prepare the ingredients beforehand: Prepare ingredients ahead of time to streamline the process of producing smoothies and juices. To make your daily routine easier, wash, chop, and store fruits and veggies in portioned containers.

Using Mindful Food to Promote Whole Health:

1. Eat with Intention: Make mindful eating a habit by bringing intention and

gratitude to your meals. Savor every taste and take a minute to be grateful for the nourishment your food gives. Better digestion and a closer relationship with your food are two benefits of mindful eating.

2. Give It A Good Chew: Take note of the way you chew. Chewing food well promotes optimal digestion and helps your body absorb the most nutrients from what you eat. Mindful chewing also helps you feel fuller and avoid overindulging.

Pay Attention to Your Body: Be aware of your body's signals of hunger and fullness. Consume food only when you're hungry and quit when you're full. Being aware of your body's cues promotes general wellbeing and fosters a positive relationship with food.

4. Reduce Distractions: Reduce distractions to establish a setting that is favorable for mindful eating. Switch off all electronics, avoid eating in front of the television, and concentrate on the flavors and textures of your food. Your appreciation of the tastes and textures of your food will improve as a result of this activity.

5. Practice Gratitude: Develop an attitude of thankfulness for the food that you eat. Think about the path your food takes, from farm to plate, and give thanks for the life and vigor it gives you.

In summary:

Including Dr. Sebi's recipes in your diet requires a multifaceted approach that includes mindful behaviors and practices in addition to dietary choices. Adopting an alkaline lifestyle, grocery shopping with awareness, meal planning and preparation skills, regularity in making smoothies and juices, and mindful eating are all important components of following Dr. Sebi's nutritional philosophy.

As you go out on this adventure, keep in mind that lasting change demands perseverance, knowledge, and an openness to discovering new gastronomic experiences. By incorporating these useful suggestions into your everyday routine, you may develop a lifestyle that supports holistic well-being in addition to physical health by living in accordance with Dr. Sebi's ideas.

Printed in Great Britain
by Amazon

46600499R00046